TANTRIC SEX

An Effective Guide to Love, Romance and Sexual Fulfillment

Richard Maxwell

TABLE OF CONTENTS

CHAPTER 1

INTRODUCTION

Tantric sex has multiple meanings, a number of that is associated with sex.

The initial that means of tantric sex refers to a ritual, formula or spell. Tantric or sacred ritual and spells were wont to reach some non secular effects.

In this context, given techniques and sex poses won't to reach magic and trance-like effects in sex.

Tantric sex originates from sexual rituals 2500–5000 years ago from the Indus depression region of Bharat.

There are not any written materials on Tantric sex as its rituals were incommunicative and were meant to be transferred and thought from one person to a different.

Tantric may be a set of teachings and life-style philosophy.

In Tantric philosophy, pleasure and joy produce and reinforce motivation to boost one's life.

The meaning of tantra is said to be the rituals that have a sensible purpose within the physical world.

Tantric sex achieves the results tangible within the planet. Love and joy scale back stress, improve health and increase energy and positivism.

Modern sex is tantra as a result of it needs specific and habitually recurrent rituals and constant follow so as to urge results.

The achieved results of Tantric rituals appear wizardly as we have a tendency to sometimes don't focus long enough on bodily sensations and therefore the present.

This is why the expertise of Tantric sex is deeply intense and even stunning for our senses.

It is not solely regarding sex. Tantric sex is quite associate degree extension of the full tantric philosophy. Trendy Tantric sexual philosophy focuses on energy exchange along with your partner.

The purpose of Tantric sex is to unharnessed repressed energy, merge energies with our partner and cleansing mind and body.

CHAPTER 2

WHAT IS TANTRIC SEX

Tantric sex may be outlined as slow sex with the accent on body and mind affiliation.

Massage, mild fondling, touching and varied techniques of ruminative respiratory end in robust orgasms.

In Tantric sex, a duct is cited because the Yoni and an erectile organ because the symbol.

An intense mental affiliation is achieved through meditating along before and through sex.

The purpose of Tantric sex is on the holistic expertise of body and sex instead of solely on the consummation.

Tantric sex is in its core the other of the western sex because it isn't regarding orgasm however regarding the wholeness of sexual expertise.

During Tantric sex, it's primary to relax, be within the moment and follow slow touches. Penetration and orgasm are solely secondary.

Also, owing to delayed penetration, consummation lasts longer and is far additional intense.

The point of Tantric sex is to induce obviate the pressure of western variety of sex.

We all expect the sex to possess a structure of a stimulation, penetration and consummation as a prize. However, the thought is to feel the intensity of the total sexual expertise while not apprehensively anticipating the consummation.

Slow and controlled respiratory relaxes and even detoxifies the body. It additionally centers you within the present and helps you get out of your head.

Look into every other's eyes whereas hugging, rather than closing them. This helps with being gift within the moment and will increase the intimacy.

Tantric sex will last for hours, even supposing it doesn't need to. It's all up to you and your partner.

Control of energy by slow respiratory, mild bit and delayed consummation creates a deeper intimacy between partners.

All of those aspects of Tantric sex heighten one's senses and build the sexual expertise a lot of intense.

CHAPTER 3

HOW TO OBSERVE TANTRIC SEX EXERCISE

As Tantric sex is all concerning intimacy between 2 partners, the subsequent exercises will assist you get a drop of Tantra:

1. Attempt the guts breath to tune into one another. Stand opposite each other and appearance into every other's eyes inserting your mitt on your partner's heart. He ought to then place his get in your left

one and you must try and match every other's respiratory for a minimum of 2 minutes.

2. Sit face-to-face (this works higher if you sit in his lap). Wrap your arms as tightly around each other and press your body against one another. this type of skin contact promotes larger feelings of intimacy.

3. make sure you move and breathe slowly throughout sex (it will facilitate to avoid any position that you just recognize

causes you to coming easily) and work towards a gradual build-up of delight. The additional slowly you'll permit your feelings and sensations to create up, the additional intense your ultimate comings.

CHAPTER 4

STEPS TO EMBARK ON TANTRIC SEX

To exploit tantric sex patterns in order to satisfy your partner with optimum satisfaction, it is best you observe the following:

Start by turning down the lights and movement out the remainder of the planet.

Loosen your body: Tantric is regarding moving energy through the body, thus as I suggest 'shaking your limbs smartly to energize and unblock your system before you start'.

keep off the bed: this may trigger the sleep button in your brain, which, in line with Louise 'means you'll be sinking for a fix romp rather than deep affiliation and infatuated sex, that is ultimately what Tantra is all regarding.

Get comfortable: attempt lying down along with your partner on the ground and slowly begin to the touch one another, taking some time to leisurely create your means around their body.

Experiment: attempt a spread of touches firm massage, lightweight feathery touches, and mild stroke. The aim here is to heighten his senses during a slow and intense means so you're building him to a peak however not taking him all the means and the other way around. Performed within the right means this will prolong sex and your pleasure for hours.

Suppose breathing: If you discover your mind starts to wander, re-focus on your respiration. Inhale as your partner exhales and the other way around it will facilitate improve the affiliation between the 2 of you and keep your mind on what's happening.

Don't provide up: If you don't last on the far side ten minutes, try again. Buddhism sex takes time to induce to grips with as a result of what we tend to achieve through sex during a western means. This implies we expect sex to possess an evident begin, middle and finish.

With follow you'll be {able to} abandoning of this concept and luxuriate in sex doltishly regarding the conclusion still as be able to management your body thus you'll be able to delay climax and increase the strength of your orgasms.

CHAPTER 5

HOW TO PERFORM TANTRIC MASTURBATION

When it involves attempting out Tantric autoeroticism, it's all concerning exploration. I will suggests taking time to (understand to grasp) and understand your own sexual story as you follow self-acceptance with none judgment whatever.

"Slow down, take some time, create the time to induce to

grasp yourself. "It's fine to possess fantasies [or] interact in sexual imagining. Just hear your body.

There aren't any specific rules for a way to perform Tantric autoeroticism as a result of there's no set formula for pleasure for all people. What works for you may not work for somebody else, and that's absolutely traditional. It's additionally vital to recollect that Tantric autoeroticism is a smaller amount concerning achieving a particular destination (or one orgasm) and a lot of concerning exploring the various sensations in your body.

If you want to undertake Tantric autoeroticism for yourself, here square measure some general tips for obtaining started:

1. **Create a comfortable, relaxing and safe environment:**

Set yourself up for relaxation and make certain to grant

yourself enough time to explore. Lighting a candle may be an excellent place to start out. However ensure you're partaking as several of your senses as attainable and extremely permitting yourself to target, well, you. What variety of atmosphere can you relish most?

Remember that tantric is additional of AN in progress observe which will result in larger awareness of your sex versus a particular self-abuse strategy for achieving climax. The goal is to find out additional concerning yourself and what you relish as you explore. And, if that idea causes you to a bit nervous, target this straightforward strategy instead

II.   Start exploring your body:

Remember to breathe and that specialize in the general sensations. Whether or not or not you begin with a fantasy or some quite sexual mental imagery is totally up to you.

What's vital is finding things that you simply get pleasure from with none kind of judgment or self-censorship concerned.

Eliminate pressure or expectations for what you "should" be doing and concentrate on learning regarding what you get pleasure from with regards to sex and pleasure.

III. Make a gradual movement:

It is tempting to rush to your destination whether or not that's through clitoris stimulation, penetration, or another technique of sexual climax entirely however tantric is regarding enjoying the journey and understanding additional regarding yourself.

One study suggests that whereas over a 3rd of girls would like clitoris stimulation to sexual climax, the type, location, pressure, and even pattern of bit accustomed bring pleasure varies greatly from girl to girl.

This means that a bit self-exploration will undoubtedly go way. For you, this would possibly involve exploring your sensitive zones or discovering alternative ways to bring yourself pleasure, like learning to search out and stimulate your G spot. It might conjointly mean experimenting together with your fingers or a sex toy.

Focus on your individual preferences, whether or not that's looking for what they're or just enjoying the items you already grasp you wish.

IV.   Do not stress yourself:

If it takes you to touch a little bit of time to induce into it, that's entirely fine too. Tantric is concerning learning what causes you to happy and discovering the way to love yourself.

It is explained that a touch self-love has some entirely worthy advantages too. She explains that partaking in tantric and Tantric autoerotism will facilitate increase your overall body awareness, boost your reference to yourself, and assist you higher perceive your own sexual desires, that helps improve your overall sex life.

CHAPTER 6

WHO CAN PRACTICE TANTRIC SEX

The good news is that there's no unhealthy news. Anyone will make love. Notwithstanding age, gender or sexual orientation, tantric is for everyone. If you're involved that it would be demanded of you be a part of some funny faith from the East, don't fret. Tantric has religious components and a few individuals incorporate their faith however none are needed. Even atheists are welcome, since, in the end, it's concerning discovery and not any explicit belief. The sole things a replacement practical should wake up the table are an open mind and a commitment to with all respect and responsibly use their new data. In tantric, gender is sacred and to not be abused.

Another fantastic attract of tantric is that it will be done reception. There is no ought to trip foreign locations and sit at the feet of a Hindu guy whose name you cannot pronounce. All you would like is yourself, a decent dose of analysis so swing it all into follow. Speaking of that, it does not take ages, either, to try and do tantric or expertise its advantages.

CHAPTER 7

TANTRIC SEX BENEFIT RELATED TO HEALTH

Tantric Sex definitely contributes to raise sexual health. It has multiple advantages for each girls and men.

Scientific and medical studies discovered well tried reasons why sexual health improves throughout Tantric sex.

One of them is redoubled respiration and element intake throughout Tantric sex. These factors encourage blood circulation and body detoxification, each vital for sexual health.

It is conjointly tried that in Tantric sex, endocrine glands are secreting additional monoamine neurotransmitter and androgen.

The secretion androgen boosts the sensation of masculinity and reduces sexual anxiety. This could result in additional openness and luxury for each a bloke and a woman whereas having sex.

If you have got problems with erectile dysfunctions and premature ejaculations, Tantric sex could be the proper resolution for you.

The slow and noncompetitive nature of Tantric sex will naturally take away psychological blocks once it involves sex.

For women, Tantric sex helps with disability or a condition wherever a lady can't reach associate degree consummation in spite of sexual stimulation.

Shifting target non penetrative pleasuring of your partner heightens all the senses.

Feeling every other's bodies by slow touches, respiration along and easily being within the moment along ends up in fantastic orgasms.

Slow, sensual touching makes Tantric sex even additional sexy. The unrushed buildup of sexual energy will result in explosive orgasms.

Tantric sex delayed orgasms area unit stronger than regular orgasms. Therefore, Tantric sex decreases depression and stress symptoms because of an unleashing of happy hormones and chemicals throughout orgasm.

Unlike the regular sex climax, Tantric sex climax will last for hours. The most distinction is that it's not isolated solely to the venereal space, however encompasses the full body, mind and spirit.

Tantric climax is among tingling sensations within the head, arms and whole body.

Adrian describes Tantric orgasm:"There may be a ton of tingling and what feels a small amount like stretching, solely terribly delicate. There could also be a form of happy lightheadedness. Aside from that, I wouldn't knowledge to explain it. It's simply happy."

The length of Tantric sex will increase the bonding and intimacy between partners. It additionally brings the next state of ecstasy to partners.

A tip for ladies is to curtail their respiration as they approach the climax.

THE END

www.ingramcontent.com/pod-product-compliance
Lightning Source LLC
Chambersburg PA
CBHW061535250726
48657CB00005B/2238